OSTEOPATHY

head-to-toe health through manipulation

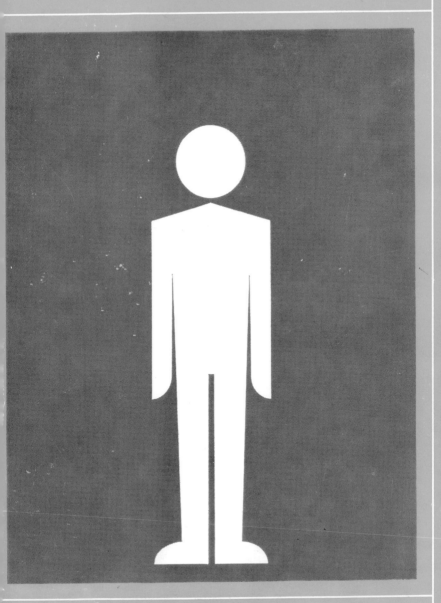

Leon Chaitow N.D., D.O., M.B.N.O.A., M.Cr.O.A.

OSTEOPATHY

OSTEOPATHY

Head-to-Toe Health Through Manipulation

by

LEON CHAITOW
N.D., D.O., M.B.N.O.A., M.Cr.O.A.
Drawings by Troy Fox

THORSONS PUBLISHERS LIMITED
Denington Estate, Wellingborough
Northamptonshire

First published February 1974

ISBN 0 7225 0245 1

Typeset by Specialised Offset Services, Liverpool
and printed by Whitstable Litho, Straker Brothers Ltd.,
Whitstable, Kent

I dedicate this book to my wife,
ALKMINI,
whose help has been invaluable
in its preparation.

CONTENTS

INTRODUCTION

For as long as man has existed on earth disease and injury have existed with him. Treatment of disease was, in pre-history, assigned to practitioners of one or another healing method. The cause of disease was ascribed, by many, to outside forces which were thought to enter the body of the sufferer. Treatment was aimed at driving out such evil or morbid influences. Others blamed aberrations within the body or soul of the victim for the disease process, and treatment was then designed to normalize the causative disturbances. These two divergent philosophies, the 'outside' or 'inside' cause, existed side by side for centuries.

In the fourth century B.C. a rational system of healing was introduced by Hippocrates. He taught that illness was often caused by quite simple things, such as eating bad food or by living in unhygienic conditions. He therefore recognized that disease could originate from external or internal factors. However he believed also that the body itself, through the healing efforts of its own nature, was the means to recovery. 'It is our natures that are the physicians of our diseases'.

He stressed that the physician should assist the ability of the body to overcome disease by removing causative factors, and by encouraging the healing effort, but never to meddle with, nor hinder nature's attempts towards recovery. Thus the school of thought that followed Hippocrates' teaching

emphasized the study of the health of man as a whole
integrated unit; relating the whole man to his environment.
Within that framework the causes of ill health were to be
found.

Other schools of thought however continued to focus
attention on the disease process itself, as an entity, largely
ignoring the patient.

The history of medicine ever since has been highlighted by
proponents of one or other of these schools of thought.
Through the ages we find the theoretical battle raging. Which
is more important, the diseased or the disease? It is true to
say that the Hippocratic concept has been more honoured
but the rival philosophy has been more practised.

Osteopathic theory is firmly in line with the concept of
Hippocrates. The patient is considered and treated as a
whole.

CHAPTER ONE
THE SCOPE OF OSTEOPATHY

Osteopathy is undoubtedly the most effective system for treating musculo-skeletal derangements and the general public has long realized this. Indeed, the average osteopath sees hundreds of these conditions each year and is able, in the majority of cases, to give speedy and effective relief from pain.

Osteopathy is, however, capable of far more effective use than simply giving symptomatic relief to sufferers of back-ache. In its infancy the pioneers of osteopathy declared that all conditions were capable of being treated successfully osteopathically. This was an exaggeration — but it was an understandable exaggeration, for it was certainly true that the scope of this system was very wide indeed. As conceived by its founder — Andrew Taylor Still — and his followers, osteopathy as a system of healing incorporated dietetics, hygienic methods (exercises, etc.), hydrotherapy (water treatment), psychotherapy (in its then primitive form), and surgery, for it was the aim of these early pioneers to find the causes of the patient's illness and to remove them. In other words, if there was a lack of harmony between an individual and his environment, the osteopath would 'adjust' the patient to his environment and nature would do the rest. This might have involved dietetic changes, exercises and spinal manipulation — or just dietetic changes, or just manipulation. The aim was always the same — to restore harmony, to allow the healing forces to work freely.

It was realized early that a great many conditions could be improved by physical manipulation — mainly of the spine. The theories that were built around many of these startling 'cures' may appear to us today to be unscientific. It is as well to remember that the general state of all medical knowledge was at that time — roughly one hundred years ago — at a very primitive stage. Not surprisingly the established orthodox medical authorities attacked the early osteopathic theories. It is still fashionable for medical authorities to quote from osteopathic works nearly a century old when attacking osteopathy. The fact remains that the results obtained were proof enough of the validity of the system.

To the early osteopath who found an immobile area of the spine of the patient, adjusted it and cured his patient of asthma, it really made no difference why. He thought he was freeing a trapped blood-vessel or nerve; he was not, but in the light of medical knowledge up to that time he was not too far out in his theorizing. Today we realize that he was certainly influencing both nerve and blood flow, but not by releasing trapped nerves and blood vessels. The effect of an adjustment is more subtle and recent research indicates that there is a 'chemical mediator' which acts through the endocrine (Hormonal) system and so influences bodily function.

Restatement of Basic Theory

What I have tried to explain is the enormous field to which osteopathy has been applied. It has limitations in treating certain conditions — but it has been used with benefit in most acute and chronic diseases.

What conditions respond to osteopathy? This requires firstly a restatement of basic theory. Disease is an effect — to cure we must remove the cause. If the cause is psychological in origin, then basic treatment should be aimed at removing the psychological factor which is producing the condition. But just as the emotions can influence the physical body, so can we, by treating the physical body, influence the emotions. It is possible, therefore, to assist the treatment of nervous and emotional illnesses by skilful osteopathic treatment. In conditions produced by dietetic indiscretions – prolonged through many years – the approach would be to correct these errors and start to build a healthy and revitalized body. In such a condition osteopathic treatment and hydrotherapy would be invaluable in improving blood supply, nerve function and, most important, adequate drainage through the lymphatic (glandular) and venous systems. In conditions produced by faulty posture, occupational stresses and incorrect body mechanics, we can again see how treatment of the muscles, ligaments and joints can influence the eventual correction of those primary conditions which may be responsible for other more serious states.

A Typical Case History

Let us consider a fairly typical case history. The patient had low back pain, aching limbs and a tendency to stiff neck and headache (eighty-five per cent of all headaches can be relieved by manipulation of the neck and head). This patient lived on a diet which contained a great deal of refined carbohydrates (white sugar and white flour and all their products), too much meat, condiments and alcohol. She was a tense and worried individual always complaining. Her posture was typical – the cares of the world on her shoulders – rounded shoulders – chin poked forward, posterior protruding. This picture is typical of dozens of patients who are having treatment from me at any given time. Her diet was corrected, more raw salads and fruit and whole wheat products were prescribed. A ban was imposed on processed carbohydrates and a reduction in meat, condiments and alcohol suggested. She was given instructions on hydrotherapy and exercises to apply at home.

Physical treatment was given to improve posture, correct spinal malalignments, to restore tone to muscles and ligaments and to induce relaxation. This was combined with a discussion of emotional problems and the patient was shown how to change her attitude to life. A general sense of well-being and relief from pain helped this change of attitude and if the patient persists in her dietetic and other home treatment she will gradually obtain a state of positive health. It is easy to observe from this that an all-round approach was necessary — there was no 'one cause' and so no simple cure for her condition. It might be added that this patient noticed an improvement in her varicose veins which had troubled her for years and was much relieved that the indigestion and heartburn which troubled her vanished during her progress towards health. In some cases, of course, results are more dramatic — but these are exceptions rather than the rule. The type of condition discussed above is common — it takes many years to get into such a state and may take some months or even years to overcome. But without manipulative treatment the result would have been far less satisfactory.

Osteopathy is of primary value in treating rheumatic conditions and all conditions involving spinal or joint injuries or diseases (barring T.B., cancer and acute degenerative arthritic conditions), especially lumbago, sciatica, brachial neuritis, neuralgia, fibrositic and myocitic conditions.

Osteopathy has been used successfully (with other natural methods), in treating many other conditions including migraine, insomnia, vertigo, ulcers, enteritis, colitis, asthma, constipation, functional cardiac conditions, haemorrhoids, amenorrheoa, dysmenorrhoea, bronchial and catarrhal disorders, etc.

I would like to end this chapter by quoting from a book published in 1899, entitled *Practice of Osteopathy,* by C.P.

McConnell — his words hold true today:

If the Osteopath is able to cure a large per cent of the "incurable" diseases, what may not be accomplished when the time comes when an equal opportunity will be given Osteopathy to demonstrate its work besides other schools of medicine with the class of "curable" diseases. For Osteopathy is not exclusively a system of mechanical therapeutics — although manipulation enters very largely into the work. It is a system that includes all methods of healing that have been found trustworthy and scientific. It takes its stand upon the principle that a correct knowledge of, and a scientific application of the anatomical, physiological and hygienic principles of human nature form the therapeutic basis of the preservation of health and the prevention and cure of disease.

CHAPTER TWO
DEVELOPMENT OF OSTEOPATHY

In order to understand osteopathy it is essential to know something of the period and setting of its origin. It is also important to know something of the man who developed it as an alternative system of healing to that existing in his time.

Founder of Osteopathy

Andrew Taylor Still was born in 1828 in Jonesburgh, Virginia. His father, Rev. Abram Still, of the Methodist Episcopal Church, was both preacher and doctor to his flock. This was not an unusual combination at this time. When Andrew was six the family moved to Tennessee, where he attended elementary school. Three years later the family moved to Northern Missouri, Abram Still having been appointed as Methodist missionary to the area. There Andrew attended a typical frontier school.

During this period Andrew displayed a great interest in the natural environment. With his father's aid he studied and observed nature. He found great beauty and symmetry in the world, marred only by the constant presence of death and disease. He was horrified by the havoc wrought by the common diseases of the day, such as smallpox, cholera and meningitis. He was sensitive to the inadequacy of current medical methods in dealing with these diseases. When Andrew was sixteen the family moved to Kansas where his father had been appointed missionary to the Shawnee Indians. At the age of eighteen Andrew Still married. In 1857 he was elected to the Kansas legislature where he promoted the anti-slavery cause. His wife died in 1859 leaving him with three young children, and he remarried in 1860. His medical training began when he was able to help and learn from his father. This apprentice system was common practice in frontier areas during this period. Before the civil war he attended the College of Physicians and Surgeons in Kansas City, but before completing the course he enlisted in the army. During the civil war he served as a surgeon and rose to the rank of major.

Following the war he continued to study the nature of health and disease. He found current theory and practice inadequate in dealing with the ravages of disease.

He studied the human body in detail, its structure and the relationship between structure and function. He became convinced that only through the understanding of the vital connection between structure and function could an answer be found to malfunctions of the body, i.e., disease.

In 1864 an epidemic of meningitis struck the Missouri frontier. Thousands died, including his three children. It was his helplessness during this tragedy that drove him on in his studies. By 1874 he considered his concepts were ready for presentation to the medical world. He had come to the belief that man should be treated as a whole, that he cannot get sick in one area of his body without involvement of other parts or organs.

Clinical Experience

The concepts and theories were proved in his clinical experience. He developed the art of manipulative therapy, based on his detailed knowledge of human anatomy, physiology and chemistry and above all on his new-found discovery of the vital inter-relationship between the structure of the body and its function.

At this time Dr Still was living in Kirksville, Missouri, his fame spread rapidly and patients came to him from all over America.

He found that by careful palpation, i.e., examination by feeling the surface of the body, he could ascertain abnormalities, and by careful manipulation he could often restore normal function. In many cases he found that he was able to achieve results where previously he had failed. He records success with pneumonia, asthma and many of the chronic diseases.

He was undoubtedly a gifted healer, and his manipulative skill was legendary. He gives details of a case of a dislocated elbow that four doctors had failed to reduce even under anaesthesia, which he reduced in minutes without an anaesthetic.

His contribution was therefore primarily to offer an alternative to the violent drugging of orthodox medicine of that time. Secondly, he not only conceived the basic theories of this new approach but developed and originated manipulative skills without any outside aid. A man of brilliance and dedication, he stubbornly persisted in his work despite enormous opposition from the medical fraternity.

In considering his achievement it is important to realize that medical knowledge as we know it today was in its infancy. Antiseptic surgery was only just being introduced by Lister, against conservative orthodox opposition. It was another twenty years before x-ray was introduced. The germ theory of Pasteur had only been established some ten years previously. It was in this dark age that Still worked out a practical system of structural therapeutics that has never been invalidated by later discoveries.

Still emphasized the importance of the musculoskeletal

system as a major factor in disease processes; he recognized the body structure as an important source of derangement. It was therefore also a major avenue for the application of therapy designed to assist natural defences and to repair and restore physiological adaptive functions.

First College of Osteopathy

The result of this view is to distinguish the patient from his ailment and to recognize finally that only by understanding the attributes of health can the disease process be studied and corrected. In order to cope with the demands of some of his fellow doctors Still trained them in his theories and techniques. This led ultimately to the founding of the first college of osteopathy in Kirksville in 1892.

Among its stated aims was to 'establish a college of Osteopathy the design of which is to improve our present system of surgery, obstetrics and treatment of diseases generally, and to place the same on a more scientific and rational basis and to impart knowledge to the medical profession.' Thus in concept the method of healing Still founded was a reforming one, not a non-medical system; but a system designed to improve the practice of medicine.

By the time Still died in 1917 at the age of eighty-nine, there were more than 5,000 osteopathic physicians practising in America.

Osteopathy in Great Britain has followed a different pattern from that in the U.S.A.

At the turn of the century osteopaths coming to Britain found a gap in medical practice which they readily filled. There was an inability and an unwillingness on the part of the medical profession to manipulate, and the early osteopaths found themselves fully employed dealing with backaches and joint problems. This pattern has tended to continue and to a large extent osteopaths in Britain find their main work in treating musculo-skeletal and general rheumatic conditions. There is however an increasing demand for osteopathic therapy in general ill-health. Such conditions as asthma, gastric disturbances and migraine respond to manipulative correction of underlying structural faults.

Cranial osteopathy has been a more recent development and a detailed consideration of this concept will be found in a later chapter.

CHAPTER THREE

MAN AND DISEASE

In the study of health and disease no single part of the human body can be considered in isolation. There is complete interdependence of one body system with another and of one organ with another. Man is a unified whole, biologically and ecologically. As an example one may consider the effects of a disease of the kidneys which would produce high blood-pressure and cardiac (heart) stress. All disease involves the whole body.

Man can be studied and understood only in relation to his environment. (This does not only mean his external environment but also his internal environment). In order to come to an understanding of the causes of disease, man must be seen in relation to his food, his work, his home life, his emotions, his relationships with others, his inherited characteristics and his attitudes to life.

Then study must be made of his hormonal and nervous systems, his circulatory system, his muscles, joints, etc. In this way a pattern will emerge which will show causes and therefore remedies for his diseases. There may be repeated dietary indiscretions and long standing stress problems. These negative influences require the body to adapt to an undesirable extent. This adaptation will always be accomplished at the expense of perfect function.

In the previous example one could see the body adapting

to its diseased kidneys, but in doing so requiring increased effort on the part of the heart. This must lead to a lowering of the body's ability to function at its optimum level of health.

When a number of such adaptive and compensatory efforts are required the disharmony may go beyond simple imbalance and lead to disease.

To contine with the example; in time the increased blood pressure and cardiac output could lead to circulatory distress or heart disease. Thus in coping with a kidney disease the body may break down in other areas or organs.

Basic Principles

From the basis of the philosophy that man must be studied as a whole in order to understand those factors necessary for health, various basic principles arise.

Firstly, osteopathy believes that the human body, when anatomically and physiologically sound, has a positive power to maintain health and to prevent disease. It follows that health is not the mere absence of disease but is a positive state of harmony within the body, and between man and his environment.

Osteopathic thinking accepts the Hippocratic tradition of the belief in the healing power of nature (*vis medicatrix naturae*). Andrew Taylor Still propounded the theory that when structural relationships are normal, environmental conditions favourable, and nutrition sound, there are within the body substances capable of maintaining health and preventing disease. The body manufactures within itself substances which resist and destroy foreign organisms, but if a poor nutritional state exists or there is a negative mental state, the response might well prove inadequate and infection and disease could result. It is obvious that in order to function normally and to respond to the demands of life, the body must have an unimpeded flow of blood and nerve impulses. It is in this area that the structural framework of the body is of vital consideration. The muscles, ligaments, fascia and bones comprise the musculoskeletal system. If the structure is in alignment then the joints will function normally and the organs of the body will be in their correct positions.

Any structural or mechanical abnormality will adversely affect the harmonious working of the body. If such a fault should persist for any length of time disease may ensue. We are all aware of the spontaneous normalization of injuries and strains. We are equally aware of a return to well-being after illness. A broken bone, a cut, a torn muscle, even a serious fracture will heal, whether we assist the process or not! (Of course in the latter case, healing would be improved if the area was splinted during the repair period). Thus our aim should be towards helping the self-healing effort which is continuously operating. In a broad sense restoration of health is assisted by sound nutrition, rest, adequate exercise, and correction of structural abnormalities, which may be hindering a return to normal.

The very centre of osteopathic reasoning is this inter-dependence between structure and function. A machine can only operate at its optimum if it is structurally sound. A complex structure such as the human body is subject to a variety of stresses, injuries and strains that interfere with correct function, and it is these anomalies that osteopathy seeks to correct.

The musculo-skeletal system comprises more than sixty per cent of the total body structure. It enables movement to take place; it supports the organs of the body; it facilitates circulation and nerve supply; it provides for shock — absorption and strain, and it is self-repairing.

Obviously accidents and injuries may occur which would interfere with normal function. But by far the greatest damage to the body structure is its lifelong struggle against the force of gravity. (see Chapter Six on posture).

The advantage which the agility of the upright position has given man is balanced by disadvantages. These handicaps are much more apparent in modern 'civilized' life than in more primitive societies.

Repetitive Stress

Modern man constantly abuses his body. Consider the compound effects of repetitive industrial or clerical occupations; of driving; of accommodating the body to ill-designed, mass produced furniture or equipment; of physiologically damaging footwear, such as shoes with high heels; and of restrictive undergarments; of habits such as cross-legged sitting, or standing with the weight on only one leg, etc. Just for a moment consider what the body has to cope with in a 'normal' day. Having slept on a too soft bed, the body is obliged to bend or stretch itself through the rigours of washing, shaving and dressing. Wash basins being of uniform size and bodies growing to random lengths can cause stress, even in the simple act of washing the face. The body next finds itself seated in a car, a train or a bus, and then subjected to hours of repetitive duties, either at a desk, at a workbench or in the home, etc. All this is being done on high heels or at a too low or too high desk, or in a seat too deep or too shallow, and in an habitually one-sided manner, with a slouch or stoop. It is not surprising that man has been described as 'a biped animal with backache'.

With this constant repetitive stress we can see why the degeneration of the spinal joints is well advanced by middle age and why backache, stiff necks and general signs of 'wear and tear' are the rule rather than the exception.

All this is obvious and easily demonstrable. What is less easy to understand is how this state of affairs translates into real ill-health and disease.

The musculoskeletal system is intimately connected with

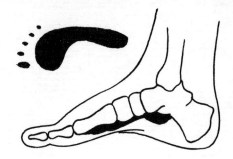

Side view of normal foot

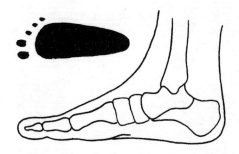

Side view of foot showing dropped arch

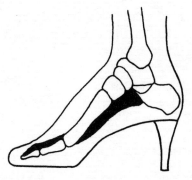

Side view of the effect on the foot of wearing high heels

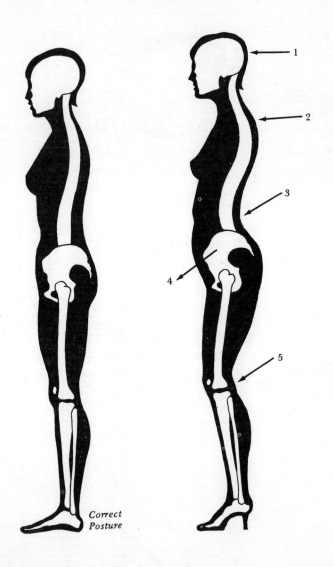

Correct Posture

The Effect of Wearing High Heels
1. Head forward of its centre of gravity 2. Thoracic area of spine rounded 3. Lumbar area hollowed 4. Pelvis rotated forward and abdominal area sagging 5. Shortening of posterior leg muscles

the other body systems through the nervous system. Changes in the nervous system are closely connected with changes in glandular function. So interdependent are these systems that changes in one lead to changes in the other and they are often considered together as the neuroendocrine system. The organs and systems of the human body are further interconnected by the relationship between the circulatory system and the neuroendocrine system.

If mechanical disorder, caused by injury, postural stress or congenital factors, exist, it is not unreasonable to expect that such problems could be transmitted through the neuroendocrine and circulatory systems, to affect other areas of the body.

Osteopathic Lesions

Disturbances so produced may be local or remote in their effects. We term these changes osteopathic lesions. These processes are observed in the muscles and joints but their effects may be found in all organs and systems. The signs may be observed in the area of the lesion or, as has been shown by recent research, the effects of the osteopathic lesion may be seen in any tissue of the body.

The human body is never static. The life process is a continual complex series of activities. There are constant balancing and adaptive processes coping with external factors such as temperature changes, energy requirements and so on. There are also constantly changing internal demands which require adaptation of one system or another to deal with the fluctuations in internal activity, and when the adaptive mechanisms can cope with the demands placed upon them, one can say that harmony between the body systems exists. With the normal ageing process the ability of the body to maintain balance decreases.

There may be an increase in nerve impulses (an amplific-

Distribution of Segmental Nerves

e.g., If the roots of 1st sacral nerve are compressed pain is felt on outside of foot (the areas indicated are supplied by the nerves from the spinal level indicated by letter and number)

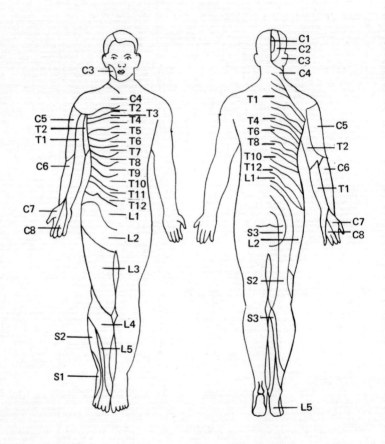

C=Cervical
T=Thoracic
L=Lumbar
S=Sacral

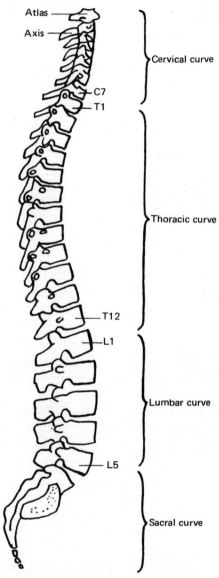

Side view of a normal spine showing the natural curves

ation of the normal impulses) due to a process known as facilitation. This may be a direct result of imbalance in the muscles or joints, or injury. There might also be a modification in nervous communication within the body in the opposite direction, a damping down or inhibiting effect. This can also be a direct result of imbalance of muscles or joints, i.e., osteopathic lesions.

Thus it should now be evident that since body health is dependent on the balanced co-operation of all the organs and systems of the body, and since this harmony is dependent on normal nerve impulses and circulation for communication, and since the vast musculoskeletal system is capable, when itself imbalanced, of disrupting or altering these systems, the so called osteopathic lesion is capable of being a major cause of ill-health, and its correction a vital factor in remedying this situation.

As an example of the inter-relationship of the body systems and the ability of a musculoskeletal lesion to produce disease, let us consider certain forms of asthma. The causes of asthma are often considered to be allergic or emotional factors. All drug treatment of asthma is dependent on the nervous and circulatory systems for its effects. It has often been found, by osteopaths, that areas of irritation within the musculoskeletal system can disturb the nervous or circulatory system, which, combined with allergic or emotional factors, can produce an asthmatic attack. In such cases carefully applied manipulative treatment can relieve an asthmatic attack. Further, by correction of these lesion areas, further attacks can often be prevented. This is not to say that the sole cause of asthma is an osteopathic lesion, but combined with other factors it is often involved in such conditions.

I would like the reader to consider the view of a group of eminent American medical specialists, Goldthwait, Brown, Swain, and Kuhns. These researchers published a study entitled *Essentials of Body Mechanics* (published by J.B.

Lippencott Co.). They attacked the apathy of the medical profession in its attitude to the study of body mechanics and go on to state:

Not only is little attention paid to differences in structure but practically no consideration is given to what happens to the function of the various organs when the easily demonstrable malposition of them is considered. With an automobile the proper running of the engine depends upon the right mixture. Too rich a mixture, the engine stalls, too thin a mixture, it stalls. Is it not possible that much of what concerns chronic medicine has to do with the imperfect functioning of sagged or misplaced organs? Is it not possible that such sagging results in imperfect general secretions, which at first are purely functional but if long continued may produce actual pathology? It seems to us that in a better understanding of structure and physiology of the individual and in a broader knowledge of the changing physiology that should be part of the varying mechanics of the body, the solution of the problems of chronic disease is largely to be found. It would seem to us to be a matter of common sense to expect health with the body so poised, or balanced, that all the organs are in their proper position and the muscles in proper balance!

This is the selfsame message that the osteopathic profession has proclaimed for so many years.

Although Andrew Taylor Still was the first to state that structure and function were totally inter-related in the economy of the human body, earlier work pointed to the same fact on a cellular level. In 1855 Virchow, the great German scientist, wrote: 'All diseases are in the last analysis reducible to disturbances, either active or passive, of large or small groups of living units, whose functional capacity is altered in accordance with the state of their molecular composition and is thus dependent on the physical and chemical changes of their content'.

In other words, pathological changes in the structure of a cell could be taken as an indication of altered function and functional capacity; conversely, an alteration in the cell's structural integrity would be the cause of altered cell function.

Osteopathy's unique contribution has been to recognize

that man is a mechanical, or biophysical complex, as well as a biochemical complex. The human body is covered by mechanical laws and therefore responds to both correct and incorrect body mechanics.

CHAPTER FOUR
OSTEOPATHIC MANIPULATION

Osteopathic manipulative therapy is far more than massage. Over the past hundred years a variety of methods, skills and techniques have been developed by osteopaths to both evaluate structural problems and to treat these, when found.

There three aims in osteopathic treatment. Firstly, there is the restoration to normal of the supporting tissues such as muscles, ligaments, fascia, etc. Then there is the normalization of movement and articulation. Finally, there is the use of reflex or mechanical influence on the body as a whole, through manipulative techniques.

It is necessary for the osteopath to develop a highly sensitive sense of touch. The judgement and skill of the practitioner is the most vital feature of manipulative treatment.

If a patient is suffering from joint disfunction it may effect him in several ways. There may be limitation of his ability to perform normal movements. Such limitation may or may not be accompanied by pain. There may also be mechanical interference with vital body processes such as breathing, circulation, digestion, etc. There might also be reflex interference with, or modification of, autonomic or central nervous activity.

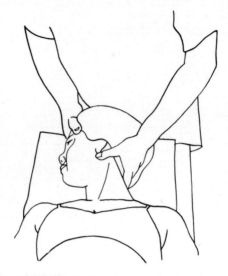

Occipito-Atlantal Mobility Test
This illustrates a test for movement at the occipito-atlantal junction. Deviations from normal, as well as restrictions of movement, are elicited

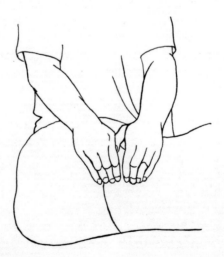

Soft Tissue Technique
This type of movement is used to relax and stretch muscles before manipulation

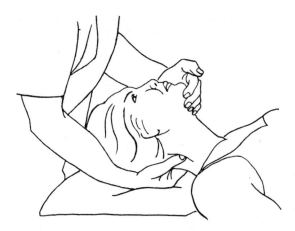

Neck Articulation
This illustrates a technique for mobilizing the joints of the neck by gentle articulation. This is suitable for conditions which are too painful for more rapid manipulation

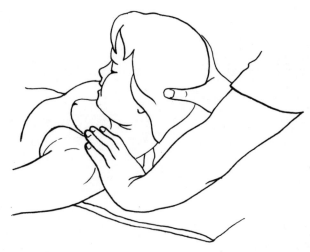

Mobility Test
The osteopath is testing the joints of the neck for normal movement

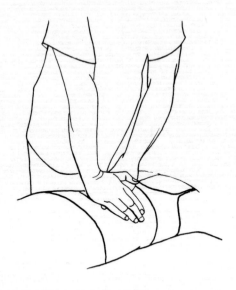

Thrust
This technique is used to 'spring' specific spinal joints in order to release fixations

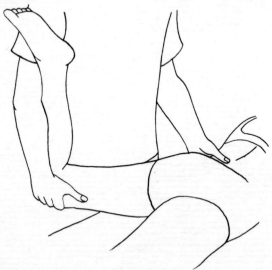

Leverage
The leg is being used as a lever. Movement takes place around the joint being stabilized by the left thumb

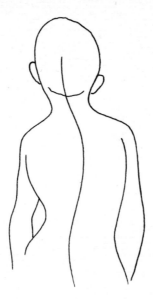

This back view of a child shows how the spinal curvature is continued by a distortion of the head

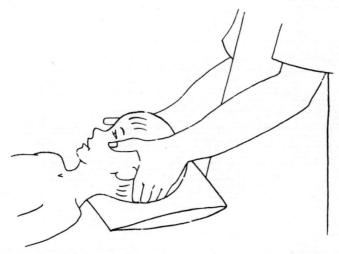

Cranial osteopathic treatment of a child

Diagnostic Methods

In testing for lesioned areas the osteopath would look for tenderness, increased or decreased temperature, muscular spasm, changes in soft tissue density and limitations or alterations in joint movement. The spinal joints, the pelvis and the cranium are the areas most likely to yield lesions affecting the general health of the patient.

Should a patient present himself with a relatively obvious injury such as a painful neck with, perhaps, associated shoulder or arm pain, then the investigation and diagnosis would be straightforward. On the other hand, should a patient complain of respiratory problems, an investigation of the rib cage and the reflex spinal areas, together with assessment of diaphragmatic and abdominal function, would be necessary. Thus, a practical survey would be made involving the whole of the body. It is quite common, for example, for the effects of a foot injury to cause a pelvic or sacral imbalance, which might produce faulty spinal mechanics and so disturb normal respiration; or should there be a lesion of the topmost vertebrae, the atlas, there could be direct effects on the musculature of the neck which has direct connection with the breathing muscles. There might also be reflex actions through the vagal nerve which could effect the heart, breathing or digestive function. So it is clear that diagnosis must be thorough. Only then can effective manipulative treatment be applied.

The object of treatment is to correct the causes of the lesion. Manipulation must be aimed at specific ends. If recurrence of the lesion is to be avoided then postural stresses, which might have contributed to the problem, must be corrected. This is not always possible, as long-standing chronic changes may be irreversible. The aim is always towards maximum functional efficiency.

Treatment would involve specialized soft tissue techniques to help normalize the supporting tissues. The manipulative techniques vary considerably. In active mobilization of a restricted area it is necessary to find out the direction of restriction. The patient would then be positioned so that the manipulation would be specific to the affected joint. The manipulative movement may be a direct thrust or may be produced by leverage. By creating a fulcrum at the point of the lesion, a limb or other part of the body may be used to lever the joint into the desired movement. The procedure may be accompanied by a cracking sound. This should not be regarded by the patient as of any importance. The sound effects are inconsequential and are not essential to the desired result.

A more gentle method, which is suitable in certain cases, is that of passive movement of joints. This method is more suitable in chronic conditions where active movements may be undesirable. A joint would be moved through its fullest possible range of motion and at the same time pressure would be applied to the restricted area. It has been found that various small degrees of motion occur in the spinal joints during breathing. The osteopath may use this knowledge to assist his active or passive manipulative efforts, by timing movements to coincide with the patient breathing in or out.

There also exists a range of techniques useful for treatment of the skull. This will be discussed in the chapter on cranial osteopathy.

Osteopathy and the Health Service

It is my belief that osteopathic care should be freely available through the National Health Service and if this could be obtained a great strain would be taken off overworked general practitioners and hospitals. The saving in lost time to industry would be enormous; already many factories and businesses refer injured workers to osteopaths, and gladly pay their fees in the knowledge that the worker will be fit weeks earlier than otherwise. Many people cannot afford to pay for treatment and this is scandalous. If they live in London there are several clinics where treatment is available at low cost, but this does not help the patient of limited means living outside the capital. Most osteopaths will reduce fees for the needy but many patients are too proud to ask.

Only by constant pressure on M.P.'s will this essential situation be reached. It will not benefit the osteopath, who is already over-worked, but it is simple justice for the overtaxed public.

I would always suggest to anyone considering consulting an osteopath that he informs his medical practitioner of his intention. In my experience there is unlikely to be any strong objection, and as the two professions each learn to appreciate the contribution that the other can make to the patient's well-being, so the ultimate benefit will be to the patient's health, and this is as it should be.

Osteopathic care is more than just the putting right of joint problems. It is also very much a system of preventive medicine. By normalizing spinal and joint irregularities before they have produced obvious symptoms an enormous amount of suffering can be avoided. Thus, many people visit osteopaths for regular 'maintenance' treatment. It is becoming more common for parents to consult osteopaths regarding their children and this is rewarding to both the osteopath and the young patient. Only when osteopathy is freely available to all will the spinal aches and pains and all the myriad joint problems of the nation be cared for adequately.

Other Forms of Manipulation

In order to appreciate the individuality of osteopathic manipulation it is necessary to consider briefly the other methods with which it is sometimes confused.

From the beginning of time the hands of the medicine-man have played a vital part in treating the sick. It is a natural instinct to rub or grasp areas of discomfort.

In many ancient systems of medicine, massage was widely used. Records of Chinese medicine dating back over 4,000 years indicate its importance even then. Massage and manipulation were used in both the Greek and the Roman civilizations.

Swedish massage was developed in the early nineteenth-century by P.H. Ling. He founded a school of medical gymnastics and promoted the use of scientific massage.

Other developments during the last century took place in Germany where the use of massage achieved great popularity.

In England there was for many centuries a tradition of 'bonesetters'. Many of these undoubtedly skilled practitioners had no formal medical training. In the early eighteenth-century a Mrs Mapp achieved a great following and was consulted by many doctors.

In 1867 Sir James Paget, an eminent physician, warned his fellow doctors, 'Few of you are likely to practice without having a bonesetter for a rival; and if he can cure a case which you have failed to cure, his fortune will be made and yours marred'.

The fame of Herbert Barker, an unqualified bonesetter, was so great that he was eventually knighted for his services. He was hounded by orthodox medicine and all contact between Barker and doctors was forbidden on pain of expulsion from the profession; this, despite his continual stream of succesful cases. In his old age Barker demonstrated his techniques to a group of orthopaedic surgeons in London, a final admission of his genius.

Manipulation as practised by bonesetters and masseurs was a relatively simple matter of pushing or pulling restricted joints, to achieve ease of movement. Sometimes great force was used and frequently damage was caused by excessive violence.

Manipulation as used by physiotherapists and orthopaedic surgeons is a great deal more refined. Nevertheless few such practitioners achieve the skill that comes with years of continuous application of manipulative techniques. Thus, when using manipulative procedures, many orthopaedic surgeons will only proceed if the patient is under an anaesthetic. The disadvantage of this is that with a totally relaxed body there is no natural resistance to guide the practitioner. Many patients are therefore over-manipulated and results are often disappointing. There has been an attempt to teach physiotherapists the rudiments of manipulation. Unfortunately they are required to treat patients only on instruction from a medical practitioner; in most cases doctors are not familiar with musculoskeletal disorders and therefore are unable to guide the physiotherapist adequately.

Recently there has been a determined effort by a group of medically qualified osteopaths to raise the standard of knowledge of their fellow medical practitioners. They have formed the Association of Manipulative Medicine and have conducted seminars and weekend courses for doctors. Many young doctors are therefore in a better position to handle common musculoskeletal problems than before.

Chiropractic is another form of manipulative treatment. It differs from osteopathy in theory as well as practice. Whereas osteopathy sees the causes of ill-health as being varied and aims to remove these causes, chiropractic theory assumes direct pressure on a nerve, by a misplaced spinal joint, to be the cause of most ill-health. The techniques are different in that chiropractic manipulation usually avoids the preliminary soft tissue loosening up (muscles, ligaments, etc.), by the osteopath, and is applied by a series of quick and specific thrusts to the affected joints.

Chiropractic treatment is effective in dealing with injuries and strains of the back. It is important to realize however the different approach of osteopathy and chiropractic to questions of general ill-health. It is true to say that the two professions have borrowed extensively from each other in techniques but that their theories are far apart.

CHAPTER FIVE
'SLIPPED DISCS'

The way we use ourselves in performing the tasks of everyday life to a large extent determines our health. The posture we adopt in our formative years tends to stay with us throughout life. It appears that we are unable to know how to carry ourselves, and use ourselves correctly. What feels right is often, demonstrably, wrong.

The effect of many years of wrong use is to produce deterioration of the spinal joints relatively early in life. Most human spines show degenerative changes before the age of thirty-five. The incidence of arthritic changes in the joints of the supporting structures, i.e., hips, knees and feet, is widespread by middle age. There are of course inherited tendencies involved in these degenerative processes. However our daily habits can aggravate or minimize these tendencies. The spinal disc is much misused.

Pain in the lower back can result from a number of causes. Muscular strain, injury, sacro-iliac strain, reflex pain from internal disease, osteo-arthritis of the spine and prolapsed intervertebral disc (P.I.D.), can all produce very similar pain. Is it any wonder that the accurate diagnosis of the cause is not easy?

Very few doctors have studied the mechanics of the spine with the degree of detail required of the qualified osteopath. The most common diagnosis given in cases of acute low back

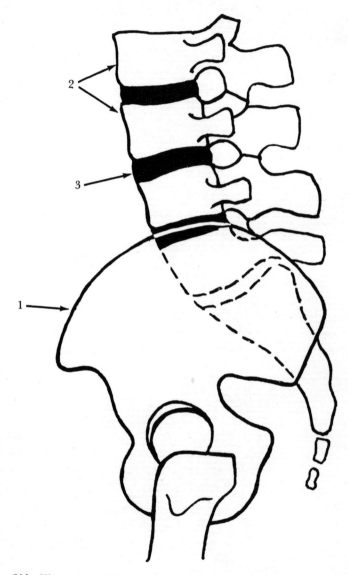

Side View of: 1. Pelvis; 2. Lumbar Vertebra Showing; 3. Inter Vertebral Discs in good position

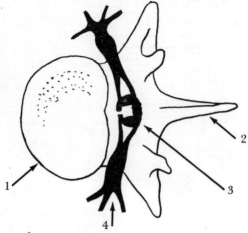

Vertebrae from above
1. Showing: 1. Vertebral Body; 2. Spinal Process; 3. Spinal Cord; 4. Branching Nerves

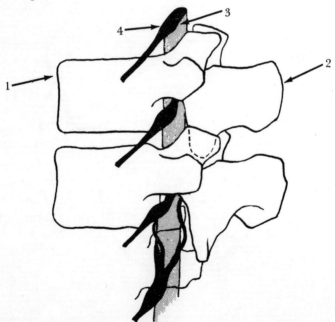

Side View of Interlocked Vertebrae
Showing: 1. Vertebral Body; 2. Spinal Process; 3. Spinal Cord; 4. Branching Nerves

pain is that of a 'slipped disc.' The symptoms vary, but usually involve stabbing pain on movement, and often one-sided spasm of the lumbar muscles; there is great difficulty in standing erect, and there may be pain down one or both legs. These symptoms are usually present in a true case of P.I.D., but may be present in any of the above mentioned conditions. How is one to know?

A detailed history of the onset will often enable a correct diagnosis to be made and with details of the past medical history and a careful physical examination, it is possible to confirm or rule out the diagnosis of a slipped disc, with a great degree of certainty.

For the unfortunate individual suffering from a strained sacro-iliac joint, who is told by his doctor that he is suffering from a 'slipped disc', life becomes very irksome. He may be put to bed for anything up to six weeks, and then put into a corset. He may find himself in a plaster cast or in some cases an operation is suggested. If the patient is really suffering from a P.I.D., the period in bed or wearing the corset would rest the area and enable a degree of repair to take place, but if the trouble is a strain of the sacro-iliac joint these treatments would be worse than useless.

In the experience of most osteopaths, the diagnosis of P.I.D. is almost always made in error by general practitioners and is very often incorrect when made by an orthopaedic surgeon. Why this should be so is hard to understand. Osteopaths have only one advantage. This is the detailed study of the structure and function of the spine and the intimate knowledge of manipulative techniques that can help the body to restore normality.

Discs Cannot Slip

The disc that is supposed to slip is a tough cartilaginous ring that is firmly attached to the vertebrae above and below it.

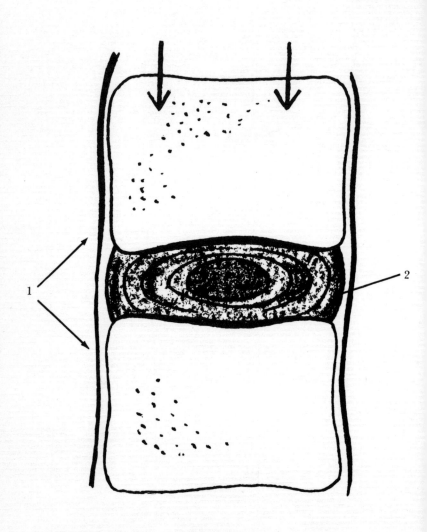

Cross Section of: 1. Vertebral Bodies
Showing: 2. Disc in healthy state

This contains an inner pulpy mass, the *nucleus pulposis*. When through strain or an injury a tear appears in the cartilage, the inner material can protrude. This will cause spasm in the surrounding musculature and if there is pressure on nerves in the area then there will be acute pain. The disc does not, indeed cannot 'slip'. There can be a rupture, or a herniation, and thus the misnamed 'slipped disc.'

The effect of long-term unnatural wear on the disc is to reduce the elasticity of the disc as a whole and to produce a narrowing, degenerative change. Thus the ability of the disc to act as a shock-absorber becomes reduced. This results in stiffness and loss of mobility and possibly pain. It is therefore apparent that anything that can be done to prevent this all too common degeneration is highly desirable.

Once a disc has herniated there is no way of putting it back. Anyone who claims to replace a 'slipped disc' is, without doubt, not being accurate. It is possible with manipulation to ease the pressure on the disc, then with gentle exercise and care the slow repair can take place. In rare cases surgery may be needed to remove the extruded pulp, but I would suggest that surgery should never be resorted to before an osteopath has been consulted.

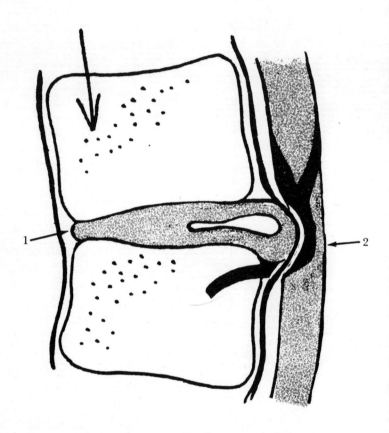

Cross Section Showing: 1. Prolapsed
Disc with: 2. Pressure on Nerve Root
Such a condition would produce sciatic pain if this occurred in the
Lumbar Spine

CHAPTER SIX
THE INFLUENCE OF POSTURE ON HEALTH

When standing correctly the weight of the body is evenly distributed. A line drawn downwards from the ear should run through the centre of the ankle bone. If it falls in front of this point then the muscles of the neck and spine will be under stress in order to support the head. As the head is held forward of its correct position there occur compensating changes in the normal curves of the spine. These changes, if prolonged, produce permanent alterations which will have their effect on every aspect of body mechanics. Similar problems occur if the head is held to one side or if the pelvis is in a position of forward or backward tilting. The problem is to know how to correct these habitual postural mistakes.

It is interesting to realize that the position of the head and neck in relation to the trunk has a determining effect on the whole economy of the body. The position of the organs of the body is maintained by the fascial bands that support them. The fascia that decides the relative position of the heart, the liver or the spleen, for example, is attached directly to the fascia of the neck, which is joined to the base of the skull. Thus any permanent deviation from normal in this area will have widespread ramifications. Once again we see how the body parts inter-relate.

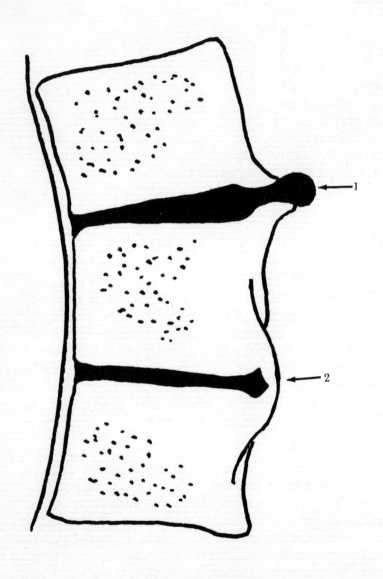

Cross Section of Spine showing: 1. Prolapsed Disc; 2. Bone Degeneration

Correct Posture

When standing, the crown of the head should be the highest point, not — as is most common — the front of the head. When sitting, the spine should be supported and not allowed to sag. The slope of the upper leg, when sitting, should be from the knee to the hip. That is to say, the knee should be higher than the hip. If this is the case and the buttocks are well back in the chair, the spine will be relaxed and supported. The feet should be so placed that by leaning forward from the sitting position and then straightening the knees, the upright position can be achieved with a minimum of effort. Crosslegged sitting produces twisting strain on the pelvic-lumbar area. It will do no harm for short periods but the danger exists of a habit pattern developing which can help to produce permanent changes in the low-back area.

When walking the head should be held 'tall', not held forward of the centre of gravity of the body. In this way the head becomes less of a heavy weight, which appears to be in danger of falling off its perch on the neck, and more of a 'balloon' floating above the erect body. Think of the graceful movement of a cat or of a ballet dancer; in both examples the head leads and the body appears to follow. Contrast them with the sagging, heavy, round-shouldered appearance so often apparent to any observer. Not only is the appearance so much more pleasing but the effects on general health and energy are demonstrably improved. Bending is essentially produced by the flexion of the knees and hips. A minimum of spinal movement should be required to get down to lift or move an object. If this could be clearly understood and practised there would be a great reduction in spinal problems.

In one-sided, repetitive activities such as digging or sweeping every effort should be made to break the pattern frequently so that other muscles can be used, and those involved in the repetitive movement given a rest.

In one's work it will pay dividends to examine the way

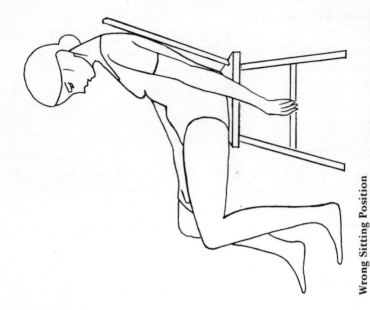

Wrong Sitting Position
Note: Knees lower than hips. General sagging of body

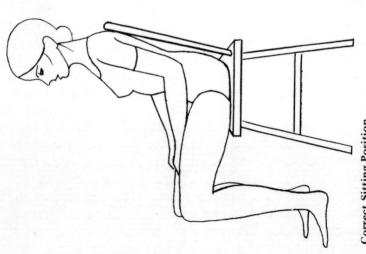

Correct Sitting Position
Note: Knees higher than hips

simple repetitive activities are performed. For example, I know of a case of severe neck pain which was produced by the habit of holding a telephone receiver between ear and shoulder, thus tilting the head to one side and leaving both hands free. This, when repeated many times a day for some years, resulted in chronic strain.

Ideal Sleeping Position

Sleep should be on a firm surface. The ideal position is to lie on one side with the head on one medium pillow which is pulled well into the angle between neck and shoulder; thus the head and neck are supported and not allowed to sag or become pushed to one side by too thick a supporting surface. The knees should be flexed so that the lower back is resting in a slightly rounded or neutral position. Sleeping face downwards is undesirable because of the effect on the low back as well as the necessity for the head to be turned to one side.

Physical exercise should involve the use of the whole body; walking, running, cycling and swimming are all desirable. One-sided activities should not be allowed to dominate physical activity to the point of producing imbalance. Exercises of a 'keep fit' nature should be carefully tailored to the individual. Yoga exercises are far more desirable as they are performed in a slow, rhythmic manner rather than in violent, jerky movements so common in the daily dozen!

To sum up, it would be well to remember that the human body is a marvellous machine and should be used as it was designed to be used. Any unnatural use may well be coped with, but always at the expense of good performance, and ultimately with the certainty of some mechanical stress. Thus we are responsible for many of our problems through using ourselves incorrectly. Osteopathy can correct the mechanical deviations and strains we produce but only we can prevent

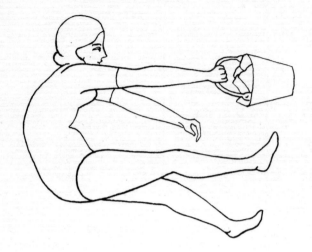

Wrong Method of Lifting
In this position the worst possible strain is being imposed on the discs of the lumbar spine

Correct Method of Lifting
Note that the knees and hips are bent and the spine is relatively straight

recurrence by discontinuing those things that caused the problem in the first place.

The way the body is carried in sitting, standing and walking is an ever varying dynamic pattern and the study of this pattern is the study of posture.

The posture of an individual is determined in childhood and the seeds of poor posture in adult life are sown in childhood. Good posture is a rarity — indeed if seen it is instantly recognizable. It is not the stiff military carriage, any more than it is the slouching, sagging posture of the fashion model! One is more likely to recognize good posture in the half naked African tribesman whose graceful carriage enables him to move in an effortless way.

Observe people as they carry out their daily tasks. Few walk well, and one is able to observe a variety of slumped, unhealthy postures when people are sitting. This is an indication of physical weakness, lack of physical exercise, and poor development. It has a direct bearing on health, both physical and mental.

The disadvantages of poor posture are numerous. There is the obvious detraction from personal appearance; also a marked reduction in the efficiency with which the individual can handle his body. There are tensions and strains that grow out of holding oneself badly and these provide a constant drain on the nervous resources of the body.

The degree to which faulty posture interferes with normal body function can be assessed by the following example of just one of the more common postural faults.

A Common Postural Fault

Lordosis occurs when the pelvis is tilted forward and there is an exaggerated forward curve of the lumbar region of the spine — (high heels, incidentally, throw the pelvis into just this position). There is a corresponding exaggeration of the

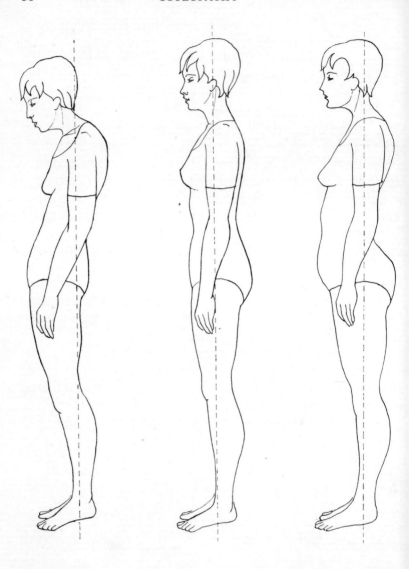

Posture
Two examples of poor posture together with one showing correct alignment. In the two incorrect examples we can see how bad body mechanics can lead to permanent alteration of muscle tone, organ displacement and stress on the spinal joints

backward curve of the dorsal spine (kyphosis), and a forward movement of the curve of the neck. These changes of the curves of the spine result in changes in the attached structures, .thus throwing strain upon the supporting ligaments, and causing malposition and crowding of the· internal organs, circulatory impediments and nerve irritation. The abdominal organs are thrust forward against the wall of the abdomen, the muscles of which become stretched under the constant pressure. The intestines and other supported structures sag and assume a lower position in the abdominal cavity. The liver may rotate forward and the common bile duct may become stretched, in some cases causing interference with bile flow. The pelvic organs are also involved, leading to many of the complications which these days seem to affect women of all ages. There is a sagging of the ovaries, the uterus is tilted forwards and down, with the weight of the abdominal organs resting on it. Varicose veins of the lower bowel (haemorrhoids), and impairment of the reproductive system may result.

With the corresponding crowding of the rib cage there is a decrease in the diameter of the chest. The diaphragm is lowered, leaving the heart in a sagging position, unsupported from below. Both respiratory function and heart action are bound to be less efficient as a result.

This tale of woe could go on for many pages, listing dozens of complaints, both of major and minor importance, all of which result from poor posture.

Osteopathy can do much to correct the damage — by relaxing tense and congested muscles and joints, by mobilizing the partially immobile joints, and by improving general muscle tone. But in order to overcome poor posture permanently there is only one course of action which must be obvious to any intelligent person.

Corrective exercises must firstly overcome the old habits of poor posture and secondly there must be the cultivation and establishment of new habits of good posture. The patient

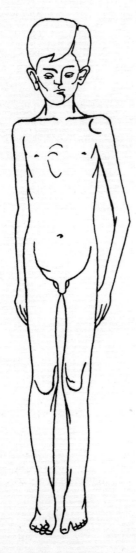

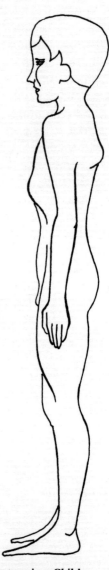

Poor Posture in a Child
Note the asymetric features, distorted chest, internal rotation of legs and foot malformation.

Poor Posture in a Child
Chest flat, shoulders forward, depression in lower chest with outward flaring of lower ribs.

must do much more than exercise — he must consciously assume and maintain correct posture for long, and ever lengthening periods, until correct posture becomes a habit.

The first obstacle to overcome is that of making the individual aware of his tension (or posture). This must be accomplished before he can begin to do anything about it. So, ideally, in postural re-education an instructor is needed in the initial stages, in order to position the body so that the patient can become aware of what it feels like to be in the right position. At first this will feel wrong and it is not until the patient can realize that what feels right is not necessarily right, that progress can begin.

The outstanding contribution to postural re-education was made by F.M. Alexander who developed a system for teaching correct posture.

Some Simple Exercises

Meanwhile a few simple exercises to improve abdominal tone and correct stooped shoulders and flat chests will help to prevent further deterioration and begin to restore normality.

1.   Lie flat on the back on the floor with a soft cushion under the head. Bend both knees so that the soles of the feet are on the floor — feet should be about a foot apart. Put both hands flat on the floor. Raise the hips from the floor a few inches. The weight of the body is then resting on the feet, shoulders and head. Swing the body from side to side (like a hammock), keeping the shoulders flat on the floor. Start slowly until you feel a rhythm and then speed up the movement so that a cycle of 20 swings — 10 to each side — takes about 2 minutes.
Lower hips and rest. Repeat the exercise.
This should be done morning and evening.
2.   To follow previous exercise: Lie flat on the back with hands behind neck. Knees should be bent and lumbar spine flat. Breathe deeply and at the same time raise the chest. Do not allow the lower abdomen to bulge or the lumbar spine to lift. Hold the chest upward and exhale by drawing lower abdomen inward and upward. Take the next breath with the chest still lifted; exhale as before without allowing the chest to

drop or lower abdomen to bulge. It is not a matter of how deep a breath you take; the important factors are the raised chest which is pushed higher with each breath, keeping the lumbar spine flat during inspiration and exhalation by the inward and upward contraction of the lower abdomen.

Do this 1-2 minutes twice daily.

3.   Lie on the back. Knees bent. Bend one knee over the chest, straighten the leg while knee is still over the chest, lower slowly, all the while holding chest up, chin in and abdomen in, and keeping the back flat as leg descends. Repeat with other leg. Repeat this 3 times with each leg at commencement and increase slowly to 10 times.

4.   Stand tall against a wall with heels 4 − 6 inches from wall. Head, hips and shoulders against wall, chin in. Stretch tall, hands on hips. Breath deeply, pulling chest upwards. Hold chest up as you exhale by drawing lower abdomen inward. Do not allow the back to arch away from the wall or the lower abdomen to bulge. Do this 5 − 10 times.

5.   Position as above, abdomen in, back flat, head up, chin in. Pull lower abdomen inward, hold for a few seconds, relax and repeat.

Do this 10 times.

6.   Position as above. Inhale, raising arms forward and upward, rise on toes, stretch tall. Let arms sink to side as heels lower. Exhale by drawing lower abdomen in. Keep chest up and forward and back flat.

Do this 5 times.

Breathing

Few people appreciate the vital importance of correct breathing. Not only is this function responsible for providing the body with oxygen but it is also an important means of eliminating waste products. The effect of respiration on circulation is not fully realized. As the lungs expand the diaphragm at the base of the lungs should more downwards to create greater room for lung expansion. At this stage the relative pressure of the lungs and pelvic area is altered. Thus when exhalation occurs, and the diaphragm rises to its normal domed position, a pump-like action is at work. The effect of this diaphragmatic pump is of the greatest importance in the circulation of blood and lymph.

The heart effectively pumps blood to the legs but in order to return to the heart, two pumping systems quite independent of the heart come into play. The first of these is the so called 'muscle-pump' system. As muscles work and perform their normal tasks they contract and relax. This has the effect of squeezing blood through the veins which, by virtue of their one-way valves, prevents any back flow. When the blood reaches the pelvic area by this action it can only move up to the lungs and heart through the pumping action of the diaphragm.

It is now possible to see why such conditions as varicose veins, haemorrhoids and other circulatory dysfunctions can be improved by exercise and correct breathing.

Unfortunately most people breath in a shallow manner, barely bringing the diaphragmatic pump into play. A further complication is that with poor posture and an inflexible spine and thoracic cage, the teaching of correct breathing is a wasted effort. However after the area has been mobilized by osteopathic manipulation and exercise, instruction as to respiration can be effectively introduced.

CHAPTER SEVEN

STRESS AND TENSION CAN KILL

The complexity of the problem of stress makes it difficult to explain in a way that will be easily understood by the layman.

By 'stress' in this context, we are talking about non-specific harmful stimuli (e.g., chronically sustained hostile tendencies; prolonged fear, unhealthy states such as jealousy, etc.). These stimuli trigger off a process which evolves through various stages. Initially a release of destructive (catabolic) substances takes place in the tissues; during this phase such symptoms as tachycardia, poor muscle tone, gastric ulcer, acidosis and many more may appear. There is then an effort on the part of the body to normalize the situation and hormones from the adrenal cortex are released to raise its resistance. During this phase there are complicated glandular changes involving the adrenal cortex, thymus and other glands. Most of the symptoms that first appeared now disappear. If the harmful stimuli continue (hate, jealousy, fear, etc.), the third and most damaging stage is reached. The original symptoms reappear and eventually death ensues.

Diseases of Adaptation

Dr Selye, who has devoted years of research to the whole

problem of stress, maintains that as a result of prolonged stress and the excessive amounts of adrenal cortical hormones produced as a defence against the effects of stress, such conditions as high blood pressure, kidney disease, heart lesions and arthritis may appear. These derangements he calls 'diseases of adaptation'.

We can begin to see, therefore, the complex interplay by which the human organism adapts itself to stress.

The problem posed by this whole complex of emotions and their destructive end products is very real for any practitioner — medical or unorthodox. Osteopaths utilize various methods of treatment, which enable patients to be helped to regain a balanced mental and physical state of health — (unless the destructive process has progressed too far for regeneration to take place).

Among these therapeutic measures are psychotherapy, relaxation techniques and various manipulative and soft tissue techniques.

It is important to remember that the mind, the body and the spirit are not separate entities but are in fact different expressions of the same thing. If, as Selye has shown, the effect of a disturbed mental outlook can have a devastating effect on the physical body, then it is equally conceivable that the mind can be influenced beneficially by physical treatment. In fact osteopathic treatment which incorporates neuro-muscular technique is often able to do just this. However if cure is to be achieved then the vicious circle of tension must be removed. The method most used is based on Eeman's relaxation technique. This takes into account the fact that nervous tension can only be quieted if there is muscular relaxation. All physical activities start as mental processes. Relaxation has to be taught as a conscious experience. In a state of complete relaxation there comes a release of pent-up emotions and deep-seated frustration and tensions. After this the process of regeneration can start and a return to health becomes possible. An excellent introduction to this technique is to be found in Harold Cotton's book *Relax Your Way to Health*, which gives practical instructions in relaxation technique.

In conditions where pathological changes have begun and where tensions are very deep-seated, a practitioner experienced in this system should be consulted. However for those who would like to learn a simple system of relaxation the above book will prove of great assistance.

To sum-up: emotional stress and tension can, and does, produce physical diseases.

A positive outlook on life and the ability to release tensions through relaxation are the best methods of prevention. Cure of existing psychosomatic conditions can only be achieved by removing the causes which are the negative emotions, by means of psychotherapy, relaxation, etc.

Above all remember that a positive approach to life really means living in present time — not dwelling on the past or dreading the future. We are only alive NOW — and it is to the 'now' — the present — that our attention and efforts should be directed. Learn to accept what cannot be changed and not to fret continually about things over which you have no control. Do one thing at a time and concentrate on what you are doing so that you can derive full pleasure from doing it well.

Negative emotions such as hate, fear, jealousy, etc., can do untold damage and it is only by being outward looking and inwardly at peace that these destructive emotions can be checked.

A Method of Relaxation

I would like to emphasize that the method of relaxation which follows is not a cure for complex emotional problems. It is of great assistance, however, in releasing physical tensions which are the outcome of the stress of modern life. The tragedy of tension is that, for the most part, the individual is not even aware it exists. This can be demonstrated quite easily by instructing a subject to relax with his eyes closed and allow his legs to be lifted without giving any assistance. Having raised the legs to an angle of about 45 degrees one leg should be left unsupported — in 99 cases out of 100 the unsupported leg will remain in mid-air, despite the subject's promise not to assist! On opening his eyes he will often express surprise at the fact that his leg is not being held up. This brings home the point that a great deal of tension exists in muscles which the individual should be able to control but is no longer able to. The type of tension we are discussing may not appear to be of great significance in the problem of health — but it is. As previously explained, muscular tension is only the outward manifestation of a deeper problem. Suffice to say that the ability to relax produces a great improvement in general well-being, sounder, more restful sleep, and greater energy. If the causative factor is a result of psychological problems, then obviously these must be dealt with by appropriate natural means.

The following relaxation method should be applied, preferably once each day for at least 20 to 30 minutes — if possible after a main meal.

1. Undo any tight constricting clothing, e.g., tie, belt, corset, bra, etc.

2. Lie down on a firm but comfortable surface, in a warm, darkened room with good ventilation. There should be no diverting sounds, e.g., radio or TV.

3. Lie on a pillow which should support the neck but should not go under the shoulders.

4. Cross the ankles or if this is not comfortable rest the feet, ankles touching. Interlock the fingers and rest the two hands over the solar-plexus.

5. Unclench the jaw — this does not mean opening the mouth; simply part the teeth with the lips together. Relax the eyes — do not hold the lids tightly, allow them to rest closed.

6. Breathing rhythmically is a great aid to relaxation. Attention to exhalation is of more value than concentrating on inhalation. Breath in fully, filling the lungs without straining. Sigh out slowly through the mouth, allowing the lungs to empty completely. Repeat this slowly and

rhythmically, breathing in and sighing out. Try to establish an unhurried rhythm. After about 8 such cycles of inhaling and exhaling, begin a further 8 cycles but as you sigh out mentally visualize yourself sinking through the surface on which you resting. Such phrases as 'I am letting go' or 'I am sinking and sagging' or 'I am heavy and I am falling' will help to start the sensation of heaviness and relaxation that is the prelude to deeper relaxation.

7. Allow your breathing to adjust to its own rhythm, it should no longer be controlled. Whether you find yourself breathing shallowly with an occasional deep breath, or whether you continue as when you were controlling the breathing, simply allow your breathing to control itself.

8. Begin to visualize the various areas of the body in sequence, e.g., neck, shoulders and arms, hands, back, abdomen, legs, feet. Do not try to do anything or to make anything happen. Try to see these areas in a state of relaxation, completely limp and lifeless.

9. If at any stage you find yourself thinking about outside factors substitute thoughts of pleasant surroundings and sensations, such as seeing yourself walking in the country; try to feel the sun and hear the birds. Such restful and positive thoughts should enable you to re-establish the state of restfulness and you can then progress with the sequence of relaxation.

10. Sleep may supervene. If it does not, then you have reached a state of limp relaxation. Remain in this state for 10 to 15 minutes, allowing the mind to dwell from time to time on any area where you are conscious of tension not released, or of tension creeping back. Or simply allow the type of restful thoughts previously described to unfold.

11. When you are about to end the session breathe deeply as at the beginning for 8 cycles of inhalation and exhalation.

12. Stretch fully, trying to copy the action of a cat after sleep. Open the eyes and get up.

It is well to remember that you will probably not reach a state of relaxation for some weeks in spite of regular practice, but when you do it will prove to be an experience well worth the effort.

CHAPTER EIGHT

CRANIAL OSTEOPATHY

The development of a specialized study of the bones of the skull in relation to ill-health is a result of the research of W.G. Sutherland. His work over a period of more than fifty years revealed that lesions occur in the cranium which can have far reaching effects on the health of the body. The lesions referred to may be actual structural malalignments or restrictions in articular motion which interfere with fluid movement within the cranium or with the circulation of blood or cerebro-spinal fluid to and from the cranium. Imbalances may result in any of the nearly forty muscles inserting into the base of the skull. A further ramification of cranial lesions is the effect on spinal balance as a whole, of distortion or misalignment within the skull, or between the skull and the atlas, (the top vertebra of the spine which articulates with the skull). Cranial osteopathy recognizes a vital link between the sacral base on which the spine stands and the cranial base which rests on the spine. Distortion in one leads to an exact reproduction of this distortion in the other. The various compensating stresses and changes which take place in the spine as a result of such distortions may therefore be corrected by normalizing the sacral or cranial problem.

It is important to realize that when speaking of movement between the bones of the skull it is not meant that there is gross movement such as exists between other bones, but more a resilience, a yielding which indicates normal healthy articulation.

The injuries which produce the lesions of the bones of the skull are various. At birth warping of the pliable bones are frequently the result of a long or complicated labour or of instrument delivery. Blows to the head at any time in life can produce lesions, as can heavy dental work, especially extractions.

The diagnosis of cranial lesions involves a complete understanding of the anatomy and physiology of the skull. Careful and gentle palpation indicates to the trained hands of the practitioner where restriction in mobility exists. Manipulation of the skull is equally gentle, especially in the case of children.

Effects of Lesions

The effects of lesions of the skull can be local or distant. Local effects can include visual, auditory or olfactory problems. Such conditions as Ménière's disease, migraine, trigeminal neuralgia, etc., may all have cranial lesions as their causes.

Distant effects of cranial lesions are varied. For example there are cases of sciatica which will not respond to other treatment until a cranial lesion is corrected. This can be best understood if it is realized that distortions in the skull cause a reciprocating distortion at the base of the spine. Imagine a length of hosepipe, some three feet long; if it is grasped at one end and twisted there will be movement of the entire tube and the other end will twist as well. If the mobile column of the spine is visualized in this way the fact that it articulates at one end with the sacrum, and at the other with the base of the skull, will lead to an understanding of the relationship between a cranial lesion in the head and a sciatic problem at

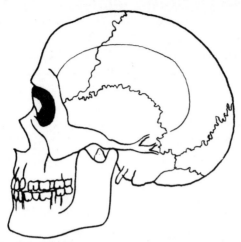

Side view of Adult Cranium

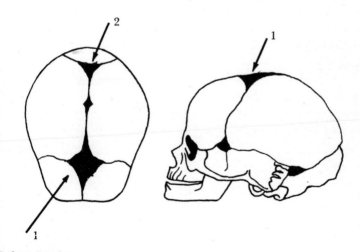

Infant Cranium
Showing: 1. Anterior Fontanelle; 2. Posterior Fontanelle

the other end of the spine. Other distant effects of cranial lesions are more complex. If there occur imbalances of circulation within the skull then neurological (nervous) and endocrine (hormonal) disturbances can also follow. The most important gland in the body is the pituitary. It lies, cradled in a bone called the sphenoid, inside the skull. Lesions and distortions of this bone are not uncommon and theoretically pituitary dysfunction can result.

Some cranial theory is not yet accepted by osteopaths as a whole; however a growing number are finding that the results achieved by the knowledge of cranial technique are invaluable.

There are several groups of English practitioners studying cranial osteopathy and an attempt to bring these together is being made by the recently formed Cranial Osteopathic Association. There is also co-operation with members of the dental profession who are anxious that their work should not result in cranial lesions. Dental work can produce problems in several ways, for example ill-fitting dentures can result in uneven pressure on the jaw and the bones articulating with it. Heavy pulling on the jaws in extraction can produce dramatic changes in the bony relationships of the skull. This tentative coming together of dentists and cranial osteopaths is a most hopeful sign.

The dramatic results of cranial treatment in many previously hopeless cases makes it the most exciting area of work for osteopaths today. No other method offers so great a chance of success in treating children with birth injuries.

CHAPTER NINE
CASE HISTORIES

In the United Kingdom the practice of osteopathy is mainly confined to the treatment of the musculoskelatal problems. Under this heading would come those back conditions often described as 'lumbago' or 'slipped disc'. The so-called 'disc' cases seen by osteopaths are in the main suffering from either lumbo-sacral strain, sacro-iliac strain or a lesion of the sacrum or lumbar spine. The symptoms of such conditions vary from local pain and stiffness to a marked distortion of the spine (through mascular spasm), with sciatic nerve involvement. These common low back conditions usually follow undue strain of some sort. Similar conditions in the neck and shoulder area, often involving the arms, are common osteopathic problems.

Benefits of Manipulation

The chronic, non-acute, spinal problems resulting from 'wear and tear' are frequently treated osteopathically. In this context it is important to realize that many such patients have been incorrectly told by their doctors that they must 'learn to live with it' or 'expect it at your age'. In fact the presence of arthritic changes and the narrowing of the disc spaces in no way precludes the chance of improvement. Of course treatment has to be carefully graduated to the age and condition of the patient and it might be that full recovery of a complete range of movement would not be possible. However even in advanced age, pain can often be substantially reduced or removed by skilled manipulation. In my own experience patients of advanced age have been told by their doctors that they could by all means consult an osteopath but they should insist on his not manipulating them, as arthritic changes had taken place. This shows a failure to grasp the essential fact that manipulation is not necessarily violent or irritating. Very often it consists of no more than a gentle process of putting a joint through a range of movement, well within the range of pain tolerance. Sometimes, indeed often, the area of pain is not touched at all. In the case of an acutely painful knee, for example, it is often possible to afford relief by treating lesions in the low back, or foot, which are causing stress to fall on the knee.

There are no joints in the body which are not treated regularly in osteopathic practice. Foot, knee and hip as well as shoulders, elbow, wrist and fingers, all these joints are treated by osteopaths for relief from lesions

We have previously touched on other conditions amenable to osteopathic treatment and it is fair to say that by improving body-mechanics, osteopathic treatment can result in a general improvement in the level of health of the patient. Thus, circulation, respiration, digestion, etc., are all capable of improvement if the structure and posture of the body are improved.

Most osteopaths rely mainly on manipulative techniques and soft-tissue treatment to achieve results. However a growing number are finding that there is much to be gained in using modern electro-therapy methods which might include short-wave diathermy, micro-wave, ultra-sonic therapy, intermittent traction, interferential therapy, etc.

It is also becoming more usual for osteopathic diagnosis to include x-ray investigation. Thus one of the main criticisms levelled at osteopaths by the medical profession is being answered.

Dealing with the pains and ills of humanity can only be satisfying if these conditions improve or disappear. Of course not every case is treated successfully, for a number of reasons. Often the patient has the feeling that results should be immediately forthcoming and is not prepared to persist with treatment. Indeed it is not uncommon for symptoms to be temporarily aggravated and although the patient is forewarned of this possibility there is a tendency to discontinue treatment. Also, of course, there are conditions which should respond, but do not. These can cause the practitioner much heart-searching and anxiety, often to no avail. If these cases were the majority it would be hard to continue in practice. One has to learn from each patient, and constantly strive to improve diagnosis and knowledge.

Many amusing incidents come to mind in reflecting on the thousands of patients I have seen over the past twelve years. Equally there are memories which remind one of sadness, despair and pain. The courage and determination to overcome ill-health is the strongest memory of all. It is, I am sure, common to all those involved in the healing professions. Not all people are brave, and not all are pleasant, but overall my patients have taught me to respect the finer character-istics of human nature. I recall with affection the spirit of my older patients — many in their late eighties. In the case histories that follow I have selected examples that I hope will illustrate something of the range of osteopathic practice today.

Female, aged 37, married, two children: This patient presented symptoms of neck ache, periodic low backache and frequent sinus inflammation, producing violent headaches. She also suffered episodes of nausea. Her history included a lobectomy for depression and heavy dental extractions some ten years previously. Osteopathically she showed neck and mid-thoracic lesions. Cranial distortion was also present. Her sinus and neck symptoms responded to cranial osteopathy and neck adjustments. Her periodic nausea was improved by manipulation of the thoracic area of the spine. Her symptoms returned to a lesser degree on three occasions over a period of six years. Each of these episodes responded to manipulation. Dietary changes were also made in this case.

Female, aged 43, married, three children: This patient suffered from left-sided migraine, periodic double vision and numbness of the left arm. She had a history of asthma and hay fever. There was a history of a childhood injury to the head, as well as a bad fall some ten years previously, at which time the base of her skull was badly jarred.

Osteopathically she showed marked congestion in the neck muscles and upper thoracic area. Cranial distortion was also present, perhaps associated with the childhood injury. Previous treatment had included drugs and hypnotherapy. After fortnightly treatment for nine months, consisting of neck and head manipulation, the incidence of migraine has reduced from weekly to approximately once in six weeks. The intensity has also diminished. She no longer suffers from double vision and the numbness of the left arm has not recurred. Treatment continues on the head and neck.

Female, aged 36, two children: Presenting symptom was left sciatic pain, since the age of seventeen. There was no obvious history of injury, and physiotherapy had failed to improve the condition. X-ray showed no abnormality. Palpation showed abnormal muscular contraction in the area of the left hip and buttock. All symptoms ceased after the first treatment, which consisted of adjustment of the sacrum and manipulation of the muscles of the area. After one year there has been no recurrence,

Female, aged 34, two children: Symptoms of pain in the lower back and right shoulder area, of a constant nature. Onset had followed childbirth eight years previously. There was a history of menstrual irregularity involving pain before the period and a very heavy loss at times. The patient was given instructions regarding dietary improvement. Osteopathic findings were of sacral torsion and lesions of the upper two lumbar vertebrae. Osteopathic treatment produced a dramatic improvement in all symptoms. The periods, two years after the initial treatment, remain normal and only infrequent treatment is required for back discomfort, usually a result of gardening or lifting.

Female, aged 54, married, no children: Presenting symptoms were of central low back pain, referred to the hip, of some three months' duration. The pains were worse at night and eased during the day. The patient had consulted her G.P., who told her that she had rheumatism and suggested she have osteopathic treatment. X-ray revealed severe destruction of the spinal bones in the lumbar area due, I suspected, to secondary tumours. She was referred back to her doctor, who was informed of the x-ray findings. The diagnosis was confirmed after hospital investigations. She died four weeks later.

Male, aged 60, office manager: The patient was in great distress at the first consultation. After sleeping in a strained position, two weeks previously, he had wakened with pain at the base of the neck. His doctor had sent him for physiotherapy. Heat treatment had increased the pain, which had extended up the neck into the head. He also had constant left arm pain. The pain was so acute that the patient was in tears whilst describing his symptoms. Osteopathic examination showed rib lesions on the left of the upper thoracic spine. Adjustment of this area led to immediate relief of all symptoms, which have not returned.

Female, aged 38, married, two children: restaurant manageress: This patient had a long history of asthma and conjunctivitis. She felt tired at all times and was depressed about the constant smarting and redness of her eyes. Advice was given regarding her diet, which was lacking in raw food.

Osteopathically she had upper thoracic and cervical lesions. These were manipulated. Six weeks later, after three treatments, she was much improved in all respects. Her eyes were no longer red or irritating; she had had no asthmatic attacks and felt far more energetic. Six months later she has maintained the improvement.

Male, aged 64, retired social worker: This patient complained of an intense aching of the left knee at night. He was easier when moving about. The symptoms had started one week previously and were disturbing his sleep.

Examination revealed no knee restriction. Palpation and mobility tests revealed a lesion of the left sacro-iliac area, with muscular involvement affecting the left buttock and thigh. An x-ray of this area showed early arthritic changes of the left hip-joint. There was also evidence of distortion of the lower lumbar vertebrae.

All knee symptoms disappeared after treatment to the low back and left hip area. Despite the early arthritic changes in the hip area, the patient is symptom-free and requires infrequent treatment to maintain his improvement.

Male, aged 84: This patient had acute pain in the right shoulder following the chopping down of a tree three days previously. He required only one treatment of the upper thoracic spine to relieve his symptoms. One year later he developed a low back pain. He could think of no cause this time, having abandoned tree-chopping following his previous experience.

On this examination he revealed a general rigidity of the area affected and gentle mobilization was performed. All back symptoms were relieved and have not returned.

Male, aged 27, industrial pipe fitter: The patient had been off work and resting in bed for eleven weeks with left leg pain which followed taking a heavy strain with his left arm. X-ray revealed no disc abnormality. Palpation and examination indicated a lesion at the junction of the lumbar and thoracic areas of the spine. After four treatments over a period of three weeks all symptoms improved and the patient was able to return to work. There has been no reccurrence.

Female, aged 39, unmarried: This patient had a fifteen-year history of acute abdominal pain. She had consulted many specialists to no avail. During several years previously she had been drinking heavily, in order to dull the pain. Osteopathic findings were of marked rigidity and lack of mobility of the upper thoracic area of the spine. She had a scoliotic spinal curve.

Her abdominal pains eased after the first few treatments and five years later have not returned. Periodic treatment is given to maintain the mobility of the spine.

Girl, aged 12: Eleven months previously the child had developed a 'ticking' noise which was audible, both to her and to others. The sound was not unlike the ticking of a clock and seemed to come from the region of the ears (both sides). She had been examined by specialists (otorhinolaryng- ologist and paediatrician) at two hospitals and had been taken to Southampton University for further tests. Apart from tranquillizers, to help the child sleep, no treatment had been given. The noise had ceased for brief periods on two occasions when the child was in a state of extreme agitation. She was sleeping very badly despite the tranquillizers. There was a history of a blow to the top of the head three years previously.

Osteopathic examination revealed a rotation lesion of the atlas (the top vertebra of the spine). Cranial examination indicated a lesion of the temporal area of the skull, on the left. During cranial treatment of this area the child reported that the noise had stopped. One week later she reported that the noise had returned after one day. During the second cranial treatment the sound again ceased. Three months later there has been no 'ticking' and the child is sleeping normally. During the period the child was receiving osteopathic treatment her G.P. referred her to a psychiatrist. He in turn referred the child back for osteopathic treatment. Recordings have been made of the unusual ticking sound at South- ampton University and by myself.

Female, aged 72,: This patient had developed right-sided sciatica after gardening some nine months previously. Her doctor had sent her for x-ray examination. When she consulted me she brought with her a note from her G.P. whom she had informed of her intention to see me. The note was to the effect that the patient was suffering from marked osteoporosis (decalcification of bone) of the spine and that he considered osteopathy unwise.

The only treatment this patient had been given thus far was in the form of pain-killing drugs. She was unable to walk more than very short distances without the pain becoming unbearable.

Osteopathically I found that she had a left sacro-iliac strain and the treatment of this by manipulation, together with ultrosonic therapy, brought immediate relief. Three months later the patient was pain-free and able to walk up to three miles quite happily. The lesson here is that the osteoporosis was not causing her pain; nor did it preclude careful manipulation.

CHAPTER TEN
OSTEOPATHY TODAY

In America there are over 15,000 osteopathic physicians in
practice. There are also some 500 osteopathic hospitals. The
status of the osteopath is equal in all respects to that of
medical practitioners.

In the U.K. the position is far less satisfactory. Osteopaths
practice under common law and have no statutory recognition.

In 1935 a private member's bill was introduced into
Parliament which was aimed at giving statutory recognition
to osteopaths. A select committee of the House of Lords was
set up to investigate the question. The end result was a series
of recommendations advising the osteopathic profession to
set its house in order. The main criticisms were of the
inadequate training standards then existing in the U.K.

In the last quarter-century there has been a vast improvement in the quality of education and training of osteopaths.
Today two colleges exist for training osteopaths to a very
high standard, as well as post-graduate facilities for the
training of qualified medical practitioners.

State Recognition?

Should osteopaths be 'recognized' by the State? This

question will have to be dealt with in the not-too-distant future. What are the obstacles to statutory recognition? Firstly there is the ever present hostility of the medical trade union, the B.M.A. The official attitude of this association is that osteopaths are 'unqualified' and therefore not fit to be elevated to a point of acceptability through recognition by the state. This argument is best countered by pointing to the fine training now offered by the British School of Osteopathy and the British College of Naturopathy and Osteopathy. Also important is the high standard of practice demanded by the two associations connected with these two colleges. The fact that there are many osteopaths in practice who have not had adequate training and are not members of professional associations is in my opinion, the strongest argument for recognition that exists. How else is the public to be protected from inferior health care? How else is there to be an honest dialogue between osteopathy and medicine, in the best interests of the patients of both groups? How else will the Government be able to insist on the highest possible standard of training and practice from practitioners of osteopathy?

If we take the position in the U.S.A. as an example, we can see that the legislation there has given the osteopaths equal status with orthodox medicine, but it has also insisted on an equal standard of training. Thus the public is protected and the quality of care is enormously enhanced.

There must be a concerted attempt to convince government agencies of the usefulness of osteopathy. The Government should be persuaded to establish a statutory register of osteopaths of good standing, just as was done in the case of doctors and dentists at the time of their statutory registration. The benefits would be to all concerned, public and practitioners.

Will it happen? Some form of Government action may result from Britain's entry into the Common Market. There is bound to be standardization of professions and the present situation is far from clear. The possibility exists that the French pattern could be adopted, for example, only qualified medical practitioners would be allowed to practice osteopathy. On the other hand the German system might prevail of registering 'health-practitioners' who are trained in a number of non-orthodox systems, including osteopathy, and are granted statutory rights alongside orthodox practitioners. The future will tell what the state will do with this problem. The question of recognition has however already been answered by the tens of thousands of satisfied patients who entrust their health problems to the osteopath.

Osteopathic Research

Various methods of research have been adopted over the years in order to substantiate osteopathic theories.

Clinical observation of the spinal condition of patients in relation to their symptoms has been carried out. There are many variables in the presenting symptoms and in the causative factors, of patients. Therefore conducting valid clinical trials on a sufficiently large scale to be scientifically accurate becomes difficult. Osteopaths individually have observed patterns of disease related to spinal conditions but other methods of research were necessary to prove these observations to be sound.

One such method was to artificially induce spinal lesions in animals and then to observe changes in physiological function and eventual pathological changes. The disadvantage of this method is that animal responses to such lesions do not necessarily relate to human conditions. However certain definite facts emerge from this type of research (all of which was carried out in the U.S.A. over the past seventy years). Various reflex pathways were proved to exist and to have a relationship to disease or pain. Changes in tissue both intimately connected with, and in some cases distant from, spinal lesions, were shown to take place.

Research utilizing x-ray has been extensively used both in the U.S.A. and in the U.K. Among the results of these efforts has been the proving of the significance and frequency of individuals having legs of slightly different lengths. The value of x-rays taken with the patient standing was also a significant contribution. This method assists in showing altered body mechanics more clearly than x-ray pictures taken lying down. Dr A Stoddard, a British medical-osteopath, has shown radiologically that various patterns of rotation occur in the spine in relation to side bending. These patterns had previously been observed clinically by osteopaths but not scientifically proved.

Various tests have been carried out to determine the effects of osteopathic manipulation on the body processes. It has been clinically shown that following treatment of the spine there is a marked tendency towards normalization of blood-pressure, whether it was too high or too low at the outset. Evidence has been collected of the changes in the blood picture of patients receiving manipulation aimed at stimulating the spleen. These results prove the value of this method in raising the level of resistance of the body to infection.

Research into the osteopathic treatment of migraine is at present being carried out at the British College of Naturopathy and Osteopathy, in London. Volunteers suffering with migraine are receiving treatment, and results after one year are very encouraging.

Research carried out in the U.S.A. has shown a common spinal pattern to exist in cases of angina pectoris. In these cases a combination of orthodox medical treatment together with osteopathic manipulation achieved success in relieving symptoms and in most cases of minimizing attacks. The result was that medication was often able to be discontinued for very long periods.

A further survey of 150 cardiac cases, some with organic

heart disease and others with 'cardiac neurosis' (i.e., their symptoms were not attributable to the heart), was conducted. It was found by x-ray investigation that 92.6 per cent showed anatomical disturbances of upper thoracic vertebrae. It was considered that this resulted in disturbance of the nerve supply to the heart and when prolonged could have been a factor in the origin of both organic heart disease or 'cardiac neurosis'. Much research continues to be carried out in America and will surely lead to further validation of the theories of the relationship between structure and function and the essential 'one-ness' of the body and its inter-related systems.

Osteopathic Training

In teaching an osteopath, great stress is laid on studying the whole patient, not just the particular area or system at fault. This is probably the main difference in attitude between the training of an osteopath and that of a medical practitioner.

The trainee osteopath studies anatomy and physiology to the same degree as his orthodox counterpart, but with a different emphasis. He must of course have a knowledge of disease and pathology but these abberations are seen in the context of being part of the complex system of inter-related functions and organs, all attempting to restore a condition of normality or health. It is the osteopath's duty to learn how to assist this effort.

The training of an osteopath has to be both theoretical and practical. At first students learn to palpate and manipulate by working on each other. Later the clinics, operated by the two London Colleges, provide raw material for further training.

It is true to say that anyone can manipulate, but not all the study possible will lead to success unless the student has a 'feel' for manipulation. The employment of skilful treatment is as much an art as a science. This is of course just as true in

surgery or dentistry, or any profession that requires manual
dexterity. The education of an osteopath lasts four years in
the U.K. If successful he may then practice as a member of
one of the two main osteopathic Associations. Both colleges
offer training quite adequate for practice in the U.K.

The emphasis on training the whole man and on respecting
the body's own constant effort towards normality, is the
great contribution that osteopathic training gives the young
practitioner. The satisfaction of the work comes with the
application of this knowledge by skilful manipulation of the
patient followed by restoration of health and freedom from
pain.

The training of an osteopath in the United Kingdom
includes the study of anatomy, physiology, pathology,
dietetics, radiography, clinical diagnosis, endocrinology, etc.,
as well as the philosophy and techniques of osteopathic
treatments. Students taking the four-year course are eligible
for grants from the County Council of the area in which the
students live. The training at the British College of Naturopathy and Osteopathy includes a wider range of training in
general health care than that given by the British School of
Osteopathy. That is to say, whilst the osteopathic training is
similar, the first mentioned training establishment puts a
greater emphasis on the importance of correct diet, and
general habits of the patient in restoring health. The letters
'D.O.' following a practitioner's name indicate the qualifi-
cation of 'Doctor of Osteopathy' (if the practitioner is
American trained), or 'Diploma of Osteopathy' (if British
trained). Unfortunately it may also indicate nothing at all, as
I have previously explained, for anyone can call himself an
osteopath. The only protection the patient has is to make
certain that the osteopath of his choice has also the letters
'M.B.N.O.A.' (Member of the British Naturopathic and
Osteopathic Association') or 'M.R.O.' (Member of the
Register of Osteopaths') or is an American-qualified osteo-
path, or is a medical practitioner who has completed a

post-graduate course in osteopathy. There are of course many extremely competent osteopaths who do not choose to belong to any Association and prospective patients should inquire·directly of such practitioners as to their qualifications. Membership of the newly formed 'Cranial Osteopathic Association' is indicated by the letters 'M.Cr.O.A.'

Glossary of Terms

GLOSSARY OF TERMS

Amenorrhoea: Absence of monthly periods.

Articulation: Joint

Atlas: The topmost vertebra of the spine

Autonomic: That part of the nervous system beyond voluntary control.

Angina pectoris: Severe pain and constriction of the chest with pain radiating to the left shoulder and down the left arm. It results from a shortage of oxygenated blood reaching the heart muscles.

Brachial plexus: A nerve centre below the shoulder blade.

Cervical: The upper seven vertebrae form the cervical area of the spine, i.e., the neck.

Cardiac neurosis: A condition in which the patient believes a heart condition to exist but where no disease can be found to explain the symptoms.

Diaphragmatic: Relating to the diaphragm, which is a musculo-tendinous partition between the chest and the abdomen.

Dysfunction: Not working correctly.

Dysmenorrhoea: Difficult or painful period.

Dorsal: The middle twelve vertebrae of the spine (below the cervical and above the lumbar areas). Also known as the thoracic area.

Ecologically: Relating the environment to the organism.

Fibrositic: Relating to inflammation of the white fibrous connective tissue of the body.

Lesion: Any alteration of structure or function, due to injury.

Lobectomy: Surgical removal of a section of an organ or gland.

Lordosis: Forward curve of the lumbar spine.

Lumbar: The lower five vertebrae of the back make up the lumbar spine.

Musculoskeletal: The bony, ligamentous and muscular framework of the body.

Myositic: Relating to inflammation of muscles.

Neuralgia: Severe pain along the course of a nerve.

Occipito-atlantal: Joint between the top vertebrae of the spine and the skull.

Olfactory: Related to the sense of smell.

Paediatrician: Specialist in children's diseases

Palpation: Feeling by hand.

Reflex: An involuntary, invariable response to a stimulus.

Sacral: Relating to the triangular bone on the base of the spine (sacrum).

Sacro-iliac: The joint between the sacrum and the large pelvic bone (ilium).

Scoliotic: Relating to a lateral curve of the spine.

Tactile: Pertaining to the sense of touch.

Thoracic: See 'Dorsal.'

Torsion: A twisting.

Trigeminal: The fifth cranial nerve supplying a large area of the face including the eyes.

OSTEOPATHY

head-to-toe health through manipulatio

A practising osteopath explains the origin of osteopathy and its successful development in modern times. Simple exercises are provided for improving abdominal tone, correcting stooped shoulders and flat chests, while a method of relaxation for releasing physical tensions is also detailed.

Few people realize that incorrect posture constitutes a health hazard. Leon Chaitow reveals the correct way to walk, sit and sleep, and gives notes on lordosis (tilting forward of the pelvis), which can be occasioned by wearing high heels. Cranial osteopathy is explained, a technique involving manipulation of the skull when lesions have occurred as a result of the warping of pliable bones at birth, blows to the head, and heavy dental work—especially extractions.

The diverse ailments which respond to osteopathy include lumbago, sciatica, brachial neuritis, neuralgia, the so-called 'slipped disc', and—more surprisingly—migraine, insomnia, asthma, constipation, functional cardiac conditions, bronchial and catarrhal disorders. The author presents a selection of case histories drawn from his own experience in treating thousands of patients, and reviews the latest trends in osteopathic research and training. On behalf of British osteopaths he enters a plea for state recognition and the granting of equal status with orthodox practitioners.

THORSONS PUBLISHERS LIMITED
Denington Estate, Wellingborou
Northamptonshire
ISBN 0 7225 0245 1

Date Due